AFTER THE FEAR
COME THE GIFTS

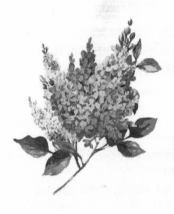

Breast Cancer's Nine Surprising Blessings

KAY METRES

AFTER THE FEAR COME THE GIFTS
Breast Cancer's Nine Surprising Blessings
by Kay Metres

Edited by Michael Coyne
Design and typesetting by Patricia A. Lynch

Published by In Extenso Press
Distributed exclusively by ACTA Publications
4848 N. Clark Street, Chicago, IL 60640, (800) 397-2282
www.actapublications.com

Quotes from Scripture are from the *New American Bible (Revised Edition)*

Library of Congress Catalog Number: 2017950187
Paperback ISBN: 978-0-87946-980-1
Printed in the United States of America
by Total Printing Systems
Year 30 29 28 27 26 25 24 23 22 21 20 19 18 17
Printing 15 14 13 12 11 10 9 8 7 6 5 4 3 2

✿ Text printed on 30% post-consumer recycled paper.

CONTENTS

◇ ◇ ◇ ◇ ◇

Preface

LET'S RECOVER TOGETHER

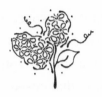

My sisters, this is what 14th-century mystic and theologian Julian of Norwich wrote in her book *Revelations of Divine Love,* after suffering from a life-threatening illness: "All will be well, all will be well, all manner of things will be well." Julian's sentiment may stand in direct contradiction to the way you remember feeling when first hearing the diagnosis: you have breast cancer. It was not at all how I felt either; it is not the usual response to the terrible news that you have a disease that may be life-threatening. This disease changes us in many ways large and small, but I came to learn that the changes in our lives are not all negative. There are moments for all of us that are terrifying and painful but, as surprising as it seems, I now see that the discoveries we make about ourselves in adversity, in confronting cancer, ought rightfully to be viewed as gifts. I have changed and grown through the struggle, not in spite of

3

it, but because of it. I suspect we all have. Sharing my experience is my gift to you, my sisters.

This book is a gift to you from a woman who, like you, was diagnosed with breast cancer. Who, like you, was frightened and unsure. The treatment process was long, bewildering, and difficult. There was more than a little pain and lots of anxiety to be endured. But now I see some very specific benefits that my body, mind, heart, and spirit received through my encounter with cancer: nine gifts—what else can we call them?—that have helped me heal and grow.

I will explain the medical specifics of my own illness so that you can compare them with your own unique experience. We suffer in a variety of ways. No two women's stories are exactly alike. Some of us have enjoyed the enduring support of friends and family; others have felt very much alone. I hope this book will be a source of comfort to all who have found themselves in common difficulty, and who I hope will come to share my understanding of the not-so-hidden blessings I have discovered.

Though your experience with cancer and mine may have been vastly different, we have many things in common. We are all women. We all have grown to womanhood in a breast-worshiping culture. Whether we are in a romantic relationship or not, whether we have nursed children or not, whether we are young or old, our breasts are an important part of our identity. We all know we can live without our breasts, but none of us wants to lose them. And we are too keenly aware that breast cancer can turn out to be deadly.

A diagnosis of breast cancer represents a major upheaval in our lives—medically, psychologically, emotionally, spiritually. It requires surrendering to a stripping process that brings us to our knees. We are stripped of certainty, predictability, privacy, and confidence in our good health. Often the unnerving news comes to us as a complete surprise. We may feel happy and healthy right up to the moment we get the news.

Just before I received my diagnosis in March, 2015, I felt terrific. I had recently closed my psychology practice and had lost twenty pounds. I was exercising regularly and feeling better than I had felt in decades. My primary health concern was neurodegenerative disease. My brother had died just months earlier of Parkinson's and my father died of the effects of Alzheimer's disease years ago. With no family history of the disease, cancer was not even on my radar. Still, as any prudent woman my age would, I had yearly mammograms. In 2015, one of those mammograms revealed the stunning reality: a tumor, about an inch long, which would turn out to be malignant.

This scenario is not uncommon. Was it like this for you, too? Many of us feel fine and happy up until our diagnosis. Breast cancer is sneaky that way. In the early stages there are commonly no symptoms. Many of us feel upended by it. It seems unreal and is so unfair. "Why me?" we ask.

My goal in writing this book is not to dwell on the dark side of breast cancer; we all know that too well. Rather I want to share the many positive things that can come out of a negative, even terrifying, experience. I have been amazed at the emotional and psychological benefits that have come out of my year with cancer. Though your experience will be different from mine in many ways, I hope that the core truth of what I am going to share will resonate with you. I hope it will increase your self-compassion, make you aware of strengths you may not have known you had, and enable you to see that, through difficulty, you can become an even better version of yourself.

I also hope that through reading this book, you will find empowerment and even joy, yes, joy, becoming more aware of your own strengths and the inestimable value you bring to the world. Most of all, I hope this book serves as your compass for moving forward with whatever the future may bring, and helps you deal with whatever comes your way confidently, with the hope and the courage our common disease can help us discover.

Understand this if nothing else: You are stronger than you realize.

We will grow through an increasing self-awareness and through examining our most important relationships with new eyes. We will find a deeper contentment when we see the real gifts hidden in our struggle. We will discover a resilience we may never have otherwise known was in us. There is truth behind the adage that you don't know what you have until it's gone.

Life-threatening illness can bring to us new wisdom about our lives—not just the big things, but even more, the oh-so-important small blessings. Mystery dwells here, too. I invite you to walk with me now through this valley, and discover things about yourself you might never have known. Welcome, my sisters, to our shared journey.

Questions for Reflection and Discussion

1. Was your breast cancer diagnosis a complete surprise, or was it expected in some way? Explain your answer.

2. How did you feel when you heard the news? What was your first reaction? How did your friends and loved ones react? How did you feel about their reactions?

3. Upon reflection, do you now see the positives of which I write in your own experience with breast cancer? If so, remember a story or two and share it if you are able.

4. Do you think that other positives may reveal themselves in the stories shared by other women? Why or why not?

Gift One

TRANSFORMATION

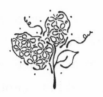

My sisters, we all have stories to share and we all have changed as a result of our ordeal. Last winter some changes became clear to me when, on a frigid January morning, I pulled on my blue down coat and ventured up the street for a walk. Chemo had flattened me on the couch for three months the previous summer, but I was finally beginning to regain some energy and decided to channel it into a daily walk. Despite the blast of freezing air as I left the house, I was determined to go as far as I could in half an hour. Striding around the block, I spied a neighbor getting mail out of his box, head down, turning back into his driveway.

I called out, "Hi, John. Morning! Good to see you. How's Linda?"

For the next twenty minutes, he poured out the painful details of his family situation. He talked about having to place his wife in a nursing home and about his son who was dying of liver failure. I stood by the curb on that winter street listening to his words and feeling great compassion. Our talk helped him name feelings that he felt ashamed about. My nose was running from the cold, but still I listened. I forgot about the time and about the freezing air and about my own misfortunes. When he was done talking and ready to go inside, I hugged him and went on my way. I left feeling gratitude for this surprising encounter. I was thankful that he shared his story and that I was in the right place at the right time to hear the story he wanted so much to tell.

This encounter was completely out of character for me. I am an introvert. Normally I would wave and say, "Morning" and keep going. But that encounter made me suddenly aware that I had changed in a significant way. After that day, I began what I now call a walking ministry, asking sincerely about the welfare of the people in my neighborhood and truly listening to their responses. The stories I hear move and engage me in ways I could not have imagined before my illness: a woman with a house in foreclosure; a young father who told me about his throat cancer; a woman whose husband had left her; and a guy up the street just diagnosed with kidney cancer. It seemed that everyone I met had a story of struggle to tell. My own story of breast cancer, also moving and engaging, has changed me forever in the many ways that I will detail in this book. I hope it inspires you to consider the positive ways your experience with cancer may have changed you.

I am a clinical psychologist and spiritual director, married, with three grown children and four grandchildren. I was looking forward to a well-earned retirement in March of 2015, when my doctor found a suspicious spot on my annual mammogram. Even though it was small, it needed evaluation. A shockingly difficult and painful biopsy was performed later that week and my primary care doctor called me three days later with the results: breast cancer.

I was numb when I heard this news. Can you relate to that? The numbness? I just thought it was surprising, and in a strange way, even sort of exciting. I wondered what all this meant, what would happen to me. I found it interesting. Clearly, I was defending myself against anxiety and trying to absorb all the stats and the range of next steps my doctor threw at me. I never expected cancer to be a part of my life story.

I'm thinking about you here, my sisters, and wondering if your experience was anything like this. Every one of us has had a slightly different, yet all too similar, experience of receiving and processing the news of our cancer. Who will I tell? How will I tell them? What might they say?

A few days after talking to my internist, my husband and I met with a surgeon to discuss our options. I felt like we were talking about someone else. This couldn't possibly be about me, could it? The surgeon was a kindly man who had performed surgery on hundreds of women. He spoke softly, but what he said was far from gentle. Options he presented included lumpectomy, mastectomy, double mastectomy, and removal of my ovaries. I heard the term "triple negative" cancer for the first time, describing a cancer that is not driven by the hormones estrogen, progesterone, or Herceptin as most breast cancers are. I was to learn this would make my cancer uniquely difficult to treat.

We also were told about genetic testing, sentinel node biopsy, and worst of all, recurrence. My head was spinning. It was way too much.

I thought, "Wait a minute. It's just a tiny little thing. Why are we even talking about this? I feel fine." It all seemed so unreal.

Our surgeon spoke as if we understood what he was talking about. I still had no idea of the significance of triple negative pathology. I didn't realize at the time that I was diagnosed with a cancer more aggressive than hormone-driven cancers; that it usually occurs in younger women or African American women; and that there is no treatment, aside from chemo, to prevent recurrence. I didn't know that I wouldn't be able to depend on the common treatment of Tamoxifen to keep the cancer at bay. All of this was so completely new to us.

Don't we become students of our pathology? Cancer makes us walking, talking experts on the topic of our disease. We Google obscure medical phrases, puzzle over an alphabet soup of medical acronyms, and struggle to understand what is happening to us, as if that might give us some dominion over it. In an odd way, it seems that it does.

We learned there are many different types of breast cancer, all treated differently. After the requisite MRI of both breasts, I had genetic testing done to see if the presence of a BRCA gene was going to further drive treatment options. I tested negative and was advised to undergo a lumpectomy with lymph node biopsy.

The lymph node biopsy revealed the bad news that the cancer had already weaseled its way into my lymphatic system. I would need both chemo and radiation.

I remember that I was in a grocery store the morning my surgeon called me on my cell phone to give me the results of the lymph node biopsy. We don't forget such moments, do we? I was holding a head of red cabbage when the phone rang. The cabbage was cold and still wet with spray. My doctor told me matter-of-factly that the cancer had already spread into my sentinel node. I would have to endure chemo. He told me that he was very surprised; he hadn't seen it coming. So much of what happens to us comes out of the darkness like this, without warning.

I was stunned by the unexpected news. When does this thing stop getting worse? I thought. Was that your experience, too? Was the way you found out very much like this? Were you as overwhelmed and dismayed as I was? Did you feel the same sense of powerlessness?

Chemotherapy, as you undoubtedly remember, in all its hundreds of permutations, is invariably tough, and affects different people in different ways. How did it affect you? The long list of side effects we may endure includes: nausea and vomiting, hair loss, weakness, rash, mouth sores, loss of appetite, edema, or the anxiety and depression they often neglect to mention on medical web sites.

In my case, chemo aggravated a debilitating case of atrial fibrillation, a common cardiac arrhythmia. I'd had A-Fib occasionally for many years, but the chemo made it chronic and more severe. The mouth sores, skin eruptions, exhaustion, and "metal mouth" were minor inconveniences compared to my heart problems. My heart was out of rhythm for many months, through four chemo cycles and thirty-three radiation treatments. At times, I feared that my heart would stop altogether. I was hospitalized twice and had to start visiting my cardiologist on a regular basis. I had to rely on others to drive me to doctors' appointments because I was too weak and too short of breath to drive myself.

When my chemo and radiation treatments ended, my doctor ordered a cardiac ablation, an invasive surgery that uses extreme heat or cold to create small scars in heart tissue to disrupt the transmission of abnormal electrical signals. (You see how we become medical experts regarding our pathologies.) But the surgeon I saw wisely recommended a three-month break to see if my heart could regain a normal rhythm on its own. During those three months, I regularly visited a practitioner of Chinese medicine who performed acupuncture and prescribed a number of herbs and curative teas. These helped my heart heal and made it possible for me to forgo the surgery.

Did some form of alternative medicine help you? Even massage therapy can help soothe our souls and calm our stressed nervous systems.

We need to explore every tool we can find to help us heal.

Sometimes all the CT scans, ultrasounds, and MRI's turn up other problems, usually surprising, often alarming problems. Did this happen to you?

One of my many tests revealed another node, this one on my lung. My oncologist feared lung cancer, which has a far higher mortality rate than my primary diagnosis. Before I could begin radiation treatments for breast cancer, doctors needed to discern whether I also had cancer in my lung. Two lung surgeries revealed that the node was benign, just a fungal infection that had grown because of my reduced ability to fight off infection. My immune system was so suppressed by chemo that by this time new growths were popping up everywhere. Seven pre-cancers also erupted on my arms.

Your experience may have been very different. You may have been nauseated. You may have had neuropathy or problems with diarrhea or constipation. You may have lost your fingernails or had any of a multitude of other problems. Cancer, and its treatment, are horribly tough on our bodies, minds, and spirits.

My recovery took a long time. Maybe yours did, too. Our bodies need time to heal and our minds, emotions, and spirits need to process all we have been through. Complicating recovery for many of us is "chemo brain," that foggy, hard-to-remember feeling that is a complication of chemo. It can last for a year or even longer, long after other side effects of treatment have passed, and plagues many of us even in recovery, as we try to piece our lives back together once again.

In spite of all these low moments, I am steadfast in my recognition of a significant upside to having breast cancer. My difficulties taught me new ways to live my life. They taught me to open myself more fully to the people around me, even the strangers living in my neighborhood. They made me more outgoing. I doubt that I would be the same woman I am today had I not endured the frightening experience of breast cancer. Anything, even any difficulty, that causes such personal growth must be viewed as a gift. You are a changed woman as well, probably more than you realize. Your suffering has made you wiser and deeper. I hope you appreciate that about your-self. I hope you are able to see, and embrace, that gift.

Questions for Reflection and Discussion

1. What was your emotional reaction to the news of your diagnosis?
2. Were you angry, sad, scared, or numb? Or something else? Have you told this story?
3. Did your feelings change as your diagnosis became more real to you?
4. Did you react in the same way you usually react to crises?
5. If you had chemo, how did it affect you? In what ways did your life change?
6. Is there anything that you would do differently? What are those things?
7. Is there anything you wish others had done differently?
8. Are you still suffering the effects of chemo? If so, in what ways?

Gift Two

LEARNING TO ASK
FOR HELP

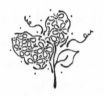

My sisters, when I was diagnosed with breast cancer, I needed time to process what was happening. Did you too? I wanted to talk to my doctors, my husband and kids, my therapist, and no one else. I tried to remain calm by staying quiet, praying, thinking, weighing my options, and trying to figure out on my own what to do next. I did not have the energy to deal with other people's concerns, field their stories about their brother's wife's cousin who'd had breast cancer too, answer all their questions, or even to hear their assurances. I just didn't want to talk about it.

The day I was diagnosed, my husband revealed the news to some friends he ran into. I was furious with him. I felt disrespected, stripped of my right to privacy.

I pounced angrily, "Haven't you ever heard of HIPAA, the patient's right to privacy?"

After I had lived with the diagnosis a few

days, I calmed down and reluctantly gave him permission to tell family members, including his large extended family. I pointedly asked him not to spread the news beyond family. He still couldn't bring himself to do it. From every corner, I had people asking how I was. Although they surely meant well, I was furious with my husband for exposing my situation to what felt like the whole world.

Marti Laney, in her book *The Introvert Advantage,* describes the profound differences between introverts and extroverts, and discusses the science of the neuropathways and neurotransmitters that drive these very different ways of dealing with the world. According to Laney, the introvert's brain is dominated by the neurotransmitter acetylcholine and has what is called a long body-brain circuit. The extrovert's brain responds more to dopamine and has a shorter body-brain circuit. What does that mean? Because of these chemical differences, the introvert takes longer to process information and does so very thoroughly, while the extrovert's brain, which gets a quicker hit of dopamine, responds to stimuli more quickly.

This fundamental neurological difference makes the two different types behave in very different ways. Introverts seek solitude to process and recharge; extroverts draw their energy from interacting with others. When I first began to process the news of my cancer, my every impulse was to withdraw. I *needed* privacy. My husband, the irrepressible extrovert, was just as powerfully compelled to talk to others. What worked for me did not work for him. And vice versa. As clearly as I see this now, I was blind to it at the time, and it became an almost daily battle.

It's unusual for me to get angry. I try to keep my problems in perspective. But when I found out that I had cancer, my usual sense of calm went out the window. I was anxious and feared the worst. I didn't want to die. I was also angry. I don't drink, don't smoke, and I have no family history of cancer. Why did this happen to me? Bad things happen to other people all the time, yes, but, to me? Even now, a year into recovery, I can barely believe I had breast cancer and am at higher risk than average of getting it again.

Talking about my cancer prematurely, when I hardly believed it myself, was difficult. I can admit now that because my husband told so many people I received an enormous amount of support: cards, phone calls, flowers, meals, visits from friends and family. I realize now that I was blessed by having people know. But at that time, keeping it quiet created the illusion that I had control, and because I felt so little control over everything else, I wanted control over the news.

Do you see yourself as more of an introvert or an extrovert? It's important that we understand this about ourselves. We can't change how our brains are wired, or how the brains of the people we love are wired. Important relationships can suffer in a crisis when we each need to manage the stress of a serious illness in different ways.

If you are an extrovert, your reaction to the news was undoubtedly very different from mine. Perhaps the roles in your life are reversed and you feel hurt that your partner or husband doesn't tell more people about what you are going through. That may be painful and baffling to you. It may make you angry.

My advice to you is to ask for what you need.

Asking for what we need makes us feel vulnerable, which is exactly why it can be so hard for many of us to be open about our needs. And sometimes we feel that if we have to ask for something it has less value when we receive it. How in the world do you make another person feel empathy? Or force a loved one who seems tone deaf to your needs to really listen? Introverts struggle with these feelings, and typically respond to others' desires ahead of, often instead of, our own. It was certainly true for me. Is that true for you too?

Susan Cain, best-selling author and co-founder of The Quiet Revolution, in her book *Quiet,* describes the struggle of introverts: they need to be protected from too much stimulation and feel exhausted by too much talk or outward expression of emotion. She also details the introvert's strengths: they process information deeply and intensely and are usually better than extroverts at detecting subtle nuances in the world around them.

Conversely, extroverts have a hard time being isolated, alone with their thoughts and feelings, and need to get their emotions out in the open. They crave social support. They more easily allow others into their world and more freely express their desires. The varying, even opposite, needs of each personality type are easily magnified during a crisis and become increasingly hard to reconcile if we fail to recognize them—and sometimes even when we do.

Many other factors influence the strategies we use to deal with our partners during times of health crisis. Much of how we communicate is learned from birth, with geographic, ethnic or cultural factors coming into play. I was raised in a quiet and bookish New England family, while my husband grew up surrounded by a sprawling ethnic Brooklyn tribe. For me, thinking before feeling is the norm, while his feelings are expressed more readily. Because I grew up in a family that didn't talk much about personal feelings, I didn't ask deeply personal questions of others in my family of origin. I learned instead to be on the lookout for pertinent clues; problems were neither to be admitted to nor talked about. A sense of secrecy filled the house, leaving my brothers and me constantly guessing what was really going on in our parents' lives.

My husband's upbringing was very different. A dizzying swirl of opinions, family gossip, and near constant chatter filled the house. At times of crisis of any kind, all parties would weigh in. Privacy was neither sought nor desired. So of course it felt unnatural to him to keep my cancer diagnosis from the family. The deep roots of our conflict—in both personality type and family culture—are clear to me now. If only they had been clear to me then.

I had other needs that my husband fulfilled beautifully. I will never forget the day he came and cried with me as my head was shaved. I'm grateful that he never blinked at the cost of a good wig and answered without complaint the daily question, "What's for dinner?" He showed his love in so many ways.

All I had to do was ask for help.

What we don't realize, and one of the important things my ordeal has taught me, is how much other people appreciate being asked to help. I found it almost funny how much my husband liked being asked. I have always prided myself on being an independent woman, and had never needed—or sought—his help so much. My husband remarked frequently that it made him feel good to be useful. Action is the best antidote to anxiety, whether for an introvert or an extrovert, and my asking him for help gave him the opportunity to divert his own worried feelings into positive actions. I learned that it is not idle talk when people say, "I wish there was something I could do." They are just waiting to be asked: to bake a casserole, run to the pharmacy, pick up groceries, to taxi us to the doctor's, to offer a sympathetic ear. I came to understand that asking for, and receiving, help was not just a gift I received; it was a gift I gave.

I had a wide variety of other needs during this early period of my illness. I wanted to get outside myself, to hear how others were doing, to focus on something beyond my own troubles. It helped me to hear about their lives, even about what difficulties our friends and family were going through. Many of us are carrying heavy burdens of stress, sorrow, or anxiety. What better way to lighten them than a quiet chat with a sympathetic listener? Such healing works both ways.

I also often wanted to sleep alone because I was exhausted from treatment, or to cozy up with a good book to get my mind off my cancer for a while before falling asleep. Happily, my husband didn't fight me on this. I expressed my need clearly, making sure he didn't mistake it for an attempted avoidance of intimacy. I also didn't want him to think I was angry or resentful. I just really needed a good night's sleep!

One of the ways cancer has changed me is that it has taught me to forthrightly express my needs and desires. Have you changed because of your breast cancer? Is it easier now to ask for what you need, or to say the things someone else might not want to hear? Does it feel less embarrassing than it used to? Are you more aware of what you really want, what you need?

I was reminded some months into my recovery of how much I have changed for the better. I belong to a church that offers a ministry to the sick. Volunteers like me visit patients who are hospitalized or in nursing homes to pray with them or deliver Communion. I was very active in this ministry before I got sick, and enjoyed it very much. As I began to feel my strength return, I decided to try it again. I was assigned a date at our local hospital and made my rounds, attempting to visit the thirty-three patients on my list. Some were out of their rooms, some were not interested, some were happy to see me. A few were critically ill and in intensive care. Some were in pain. Many were doubtful about their prognosis. I remembered from my own time in the hospital the rumpled bed sheets, the night-long dinging of monitors, the tangle of IV-drips and cords, the stink of sickness, and the cluttered trays of congealed food. As soon as I finished my visits, I turned in my patient info sheet and hurried out to my car.

I slouched in the driver's seat with my mind screaming, *No! I don't want to do this!* I closed my eyes in exhaustion and tried to release my breath. I was depressed. I had just committed myself to do this work for at least a year. How could I possibly back out on my first day?

But here's the miracle: I somehow found the courage to text the coordinator to tell him that I wasn't ready. It was too soon after all my own hospitalizations.

For once in my life, I said no.

As soon as I made the decision, I exhaled in relief. Before I had even started the car, I received a very understanding and kind response. The old me would have continued the ministry, no matter how personally depleting it may have become. But breast cancer has taught me to honor my instincts to stay healthy.

There were other changes, especially in my closest relationships. My husband began to recognize how much he expected me to do things that he could easily do for himself. I had waited on him for years when he was ensconced in his recliner, bringing him his glasses, the phone, a glass of water. Usually I was up and didn't mind, but we both began to realize that this was one dynamic of our life together that needed to change. When he reverts, I tease him, saying, "Is your polio back again?"

He catches himself now, asking me to do

something he could clearly do himself. He needed to step up, and I needed to let go of feeling that I had to cater to him. The change has been healthy for both of us, and it all happened as a direct result of my illness.

Many years ago, I worked as a chaplain in the oncology unit of a major hospital. I remember visiting an elderly woman who was dying of cancer. While I was there, her husband came in and asked her what he should have for dinner! He seemed to be completely unaware of how inappropriate his question was. I now have clarity that my own past behavior could have easily led to a codependent relationship like that. I'm glad that my experience with breast cancer has awakened me. I now realize that it's okay to just say "No!"

Questions for Reflection and Discussion

1. How did you tell others of your diagnosis?
2. How much support did you need or want?
3. Were your needs honored during this difficult time? In what ways?
4. Were you able to ask for what you needed? Whom did you ask?
5. Did you have a sense at the time that asking for help was a kind of giving. Do you have that sense now?
6. Can you ask more easily now than you used to? How has that made your life better? How has it made others' lives better?

Gift Three

INTERDEPENDENCE

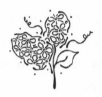

My sisters, when you've been raised to believe— as many women of my generation have—that self-reliance is the Eleventh Commandment, it's not easy to find yourself depending on others. I have always felt proud that I didn't need help from others. Consider the following vignette from my early childhood.

I'm a sturdy little four-year old with blonde, curly hair, wearing a blue sun suit and white sandals on the Nantucket Steamship. The June sun spills pools of gold around the deck, where my brothers lurch about, skipping with excitement and little boy machismo. Mom, slim and beautiful in her flowered black dress, stands beside Dad, who appears calm and happy. He smiles with pleasure as he watches every detail of marine engines rumbling into life and the casting off of lines, commenting on the wind direction and wave height. He has loved being on boats all his life.

Thirty minutes into our crossing, the air is pierced by a woman's screams. After a few seconds of confused silence comes the frantic yelling of many voices.

"Oh, God, we've hit a sailboat!"

Rushing feet pound across the deck and I feel that secret thrill of disaster. All at once, our boat tilts perilously to port, as hundreds of gaping passengers lean over that rail and point to the accident.

I'm scared and certain the boat will tip. I rush over to starboard and press my feet to the floor as hard as I can, hoping to balance the boat. After a few minutes, Daddy sees me and strides over.

"Kay, why are you here?"

"Daddy, I'm trying to keep the boat from tipping over."

"Don't you know that one little girl can't balance a big boat?"

I relax and exhale. His words both warm and confuse me. *Aren't I big enough?* Daddy takes my hand and leads me back to the family.

"She was trying to keep the boat from tipping over," he tells my mom. Humor and tenderness fill his voice.

This memory illustrates a defining belief that I have clung to all my life: that I can right the ship myself, balance the boat, correct what's wrong, and save everyone. Like most personal mythologies, this creed has been sorely tested in the real world.

The diagnosis of breast cancer, or any frightening disease, requires us to relinquish some control and allow others to care for us. We have to let others serve us, to fix things, to figure it out and cure, or at least heal, what's wrong. The need to rely on our internists, surgeons, oncologists, radiologists, cardiologists, pulmonologists, and dermatologists forces us into an unfamiliar dependency that often chafes. But we have to come to understand that what is really at work is *interdependence*, and that it is a good, not a bad, thing. Our doctors need us to help them too, to inform them about our symptoms, our fears, and our difficulties throughout the months or years of treatment so they can better help us.

We also need to rely on our friends and families, which may leave us feeling diminished. The inability to care for ourselves—and for others we routinely cared for—feels a lot like failure. But I finally discovered that there is wonderful psychological growth in admitting a need for others and learning to ask for help. Mental health professionals understand very well the importance of community support when patients are recovering from mental illness. But physical illness may also tend to alienate us from communities that can help with our healing. We may cower, like an injured bird in a bush, often feeling shame at our affliction. We hide our bare heads, our edema, our "bad" skin, gloss over our symptoms, and may be inclined to lie about how good we feel or how great we are doing. Cancer, we may feel, is a private matter. But we need to find the strength, yes, strength, to depend on others, to ask for whatever help we need from people around us. They may be confronting their own fears, and may be bewildered themselves about how to respond to our predicament in a caring and useful way. Often they are just waiting to be told how to help.

During my treatment process, I felt a need to see my children. I wanted to see just them, and not their spouses and children, whom I more typically would love to see. I realized that my life might be shorter than I had expected and I needed to cry and share hope with the sons and the daughter I had given birth to. And they came, traveling to Chicago, where I live, from Ohio, California, and Washington, DC. It meant so much to me.

Were you able to ask your family for support? Did they rally around you as mine did? I hope so, but that is sometimes not the case. Sometimes family and friends back away. Some people seem to disappear at times like these. I was surprised to see that some people I thought of as very close couldn't be there for me, while others who had been less close turned up beautifully. Some people are so frightened by cancer that they withdraw. This can be painful, but it's to be expected. People may just tell themselves they are respecting your privacy.

Many of my friends visited, called, wrote, and sent gifts of flowers and chocolate. I felt guilty for unanswered and unreturned calls, but no one held it against me. Their love was truly offered without any expectation of a response. What a blessing it was for a professional care-taker like me to be taken care of, to not have to know all the answers, but instead to surrender to the loving hands of others.

It's useful to consider the messages we re-ceived in our early years about independence, dependence, and interdependence. This can get complicated for most families. Many women, probably like you, definitely like me, grew up in families in which the mom did far more than her fair share of keeping the family and the home functioning. Some of us find it hard to ask for help. We consider all the things we do for oth-ers an important expression of the love we feel for them. For many women, getting care, rath-er than giving care, seems all wrong. It feels like giving up who we are. How often do we neglect our own health to care for our families?

Does this sound like you? I'm sorry to say that it sounds like me. For many years, exercise was something I did only after everyone else's needs were met. And I didn't insist that my kids help in the house when they were growing up because I thought I didn't need help. It would have been better for both me and for them if I had taught them that their help was needed.

In some families, like my birth family, being "needy" is viewed as a character defect. Needing help, needing support, needing advice are considered a sign of immaturity, even a cause for shame. In my home, it was my dad who did almost everything and I wanted to be like him. It has taken me a long time to see that it can be prideful not to need anyone, to think you never need help. It has been humbling to admit this. It wasn't until I got breast cancer that this became really clear to me. I was finally able to surrender some pride and accept the help that was available for the asking.

The ideal attitude seems to be to accept the emerging relationships as relationships of interdependence: relying on others sometimes and caring for them at other times. If we can get this balance right, all our lives will be easier. But early imprinting is hard to overcome. Let me share the memory of a commonplace moment with you.

It is a typical Saturday morning in 1960. Mom is putting away the breakfast things and my brothers have scattered. Dad walks through the kitchen door having just finished changing the oil, checking out the Chevy's fluid levels and tire pressure. He wears his usual Saturday uniform: old tan pants, blue plaid flannel shirt, and work boots. He is a tall, handsome man, with large hands and feet, blue eyes, and a gentle smile. He is engaged in what he does and ready for the next chore on the list: fixing that leaking p-trap under the kitchen sink. After that, he intends to climb up to our three-story roof to replace a few shingles that blew off in a storm earlier in the week. He will do all of this without complaint and without a thought of asking anyone to help. He likes to work. He doesn't feel the need to hire anyone when he can do the job himself.

I greatly admired my dad. I loved his gentleness, his quietness, his probing mind, his wide reading, and his lack of complaining. I especially loved his occasional quirky joke, told with a wry smile. He was a man complete unto himself, needing no one else to be happy or to do whatever was required of him.

He repaired the roof, changed the car's oil, repaired and replaced plumbing, and ferreted out and fixed electrical problems. He caulked, painted, and rebuilt windows, cabinets, and doors. He fixed appliances, large and small, whistling as he puttered. Instead of hiring a financial advisor, he studied investment opportunities and made his own choices. He eschewed dentists and doctors, losing teeth and risking death once due to a burst appendix, but persisted in thinking, who needs a doctor? Auto mechanics were equally unnecessary. And therapists—are you kidding? Even when times turned very hard, and Mom's health was faltering, he turned inward, never outward. As far as I know, he didn't even need God—whose existence he remained skeptical of.

Dad believed his role as a father was to be a teacher, and he taught much more by his example than by his words. When I was in high school, we would sit at the kitchen table, he with his coffee and Kents and I with my coffee and rapt attention. We would talk for hours about the economy, the workings of government, the Republican Party, the politics of the day. Through all these topics, he always came back to his unvarying motifs: self-reliance and self-respect. In his unbending view, these values were inescapably intertwined. How can you respect yourself if you lean on other people?

Even as a young adult, I wanted to be like my dad. I grew up excessively self-reliant and have all my life found it difficult to turn to others. I enjoy my friends, and of course want to be with them, and always offer whatever help I can when needed. But *me* need *them*?

Breast cancer blew a big hole in my long-standing habit of excessive independence. It reminded me that I'm only human and that I too have very human needs. The change my illness wrought, this learning to seek out and trust in others, has turned out to be a blessing in my life. Now I don't hesitate to ask my husband to get things down with a ladder, to help me understand our investment decisions, to give me directions on a trip. When I can't remember a word or a name, which happens frequently, I ask for help. When I am sad, I call a friend and talk. As soon as I became aware that my hearing was going, I saw an audiologist. I know that as I age this new-found habit will become very valuable to me. I sometimes laugh now at my years of stubbornness. But I have found a great solace in finding myself not so alone in confronting the difficulties, large and small, that life brings to me. My life is better in immeasurable ways since I learned to ask others to join with me, to come stand on my side of the steamship, to help keep us all afloat on this great unsteady boat we are crossing on together.

For me, learning to turn to others for help was about nothing less than finally accepting my humanity, my mortality, and admitting that every aspect of my life is not under my direct personal control. Whew! Is it as hard for you to say that as it has been for me? I wish that I could say that I've got it completely figured out, but the truth is, I've just begun. Finding courage, even the courage to surrender, is probably going to remain a life-long journey for me, and, I expect, for most of us. As we continue our recovery, we may find that we're more relaxed and at peace, more willing to rest when we should, quicker to laugh at our own foibles when we mess up, and more accepting of our very human limitations.

What gifts we have received from breast cancer!

Questions for Reflection and Discussion

1. How do you handle a crisis?
2. Do you depend mostly on yourself or do you feel free to ask others for help?
3. Were others available to you when you needed help to "balance your boat?"
4. Do you see asking for help from others as a loss of independence? As a burden you place on them? Or a gift you have to give? Explain.

Gift Four

SURRENDER

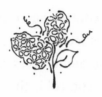

My sisters, what does the word *surrender* mean to you? Maybe it means to be defeated, to give up, or to let go. Maybe it means failure, humiliation, or sadness. Maybe it means giving up battles we can't win with our spouses or kids, or relinquishing a home to foreclosure. All of these situations of surrender are accompanied by a profound sense of loss. But there is another side to surrendering. The willingness to let go, especially to let go of control, can bring with it a profound sense of freedom.

Being in control—even the illusion of being in control—gives us a sense of security and safety. It helps us deal with the unpredictability of life. It gives us the feeling that we can manage difficult things as long as our hands are firmly on the steering wheel. The need for control underlies human relationships in every area of our lives, from the geopolitical to the personal. Learning to control our bodily functions as toddlers helps us feel like big kids. Learning to manage money as adults gives us a sense of security. Fighting for control is the underlying cause of many squabbles between husbands and wives, and between parents and children.

Our surrender of control usually comes only after a long struggle to hold on. My experience with breast cancer has taught me that learning to surrender control can actually bring great peace and contentment. When we are struck by a dangerous illness we are not just physically challenged, but also psychologically and emotionally stressed. As patients we often try to demonstrate control by blaming the doctor, the hospital, or nurse, or by relentlessly seeking second and third opinions, hoping to finally hear the answer we want to hear. The treatments we endure assault our bodies and our spirits. Feeling out of control over what is being done to us breeds anger and resentment.

When we are diagnosed with breast cancer, we suddenly find ourselves entangled in a maelstrom of often confusing information, hesitant assurances, indeterminate prognoses, and protocols for our care that are determined not by us but by others. Because breast cancer is so common, treatment strategies can seem set in stone. To the medical professionals, who have seen many cancers, our story and our plan of care may be routine. It is anything but that for us. The frightening reality of our disease at first does not even seem real to us. *How could I have cancer? I feel terrific.* To move forward, we have to find the courage to leap into the unknown, to swing out over a chasm and let go of the rope.

All my life I have always needed to be the one in control. At times during my childhood, my home life was undeniably tumultuous. I took solace in self-reliance, trying to be like my dad. But my experience with breast cancer has taught me that an overweening need to be completely self-reliant can mask an ultimate fear of surrender that does not help, but hinders us. During my treatment I needed to find a middle ground where I could ask for as much help as I needed but still maintain my independence.

As the months of treatment wore on, I was plagued by unanswered, sometimes unanswerable, questions. Maybe you were too. Questions like how would chemo affect me now and in years to come? Would I get radiation burns? Would the cancer come back? Focusing my attention on the unknown was a certain recipe for anxiety. I finally decided to surrender myself to the process, knowing I might never know the answers to these questions. In that moment of surrender, I discovered peace. I just needed to trust the process and let go of the outcome. I needed to find the blessing of simply having faith, and I did.

Why is the task of letting go so hard for many of us? Our expectations may be to blame: this new reality doesn't fit in with the way we think our lives are supposed to unfold. We think that if we eat right, exercise, and take care of our health nothing bad will happen to us. Our personality may also play a role. Some of us have always feared the unknown. Some simply resent change. Some of us take a dark pleasure in pointing out what others have done that may have caused their illness. But instead of blaming others—or ourselves—we need to find the wisdom, and the ways, to practice self-compassion.

Let's take a closer look at what we have endured and what we've grown to accept. When we were diagnosed with breast cancer, our privacy was among the first things we lost. We were repeatedly examined by a variety of often anonymous doctors, nurses, and lab techs. Not people we knew, or had any prior relationship with, but strangers who were only doing their jobs—however well they did them. Some of our body parts were surgically removed, either a part of a breast, a whole breast, or both breasts. When we recovered from that, some of us endured yet another surgery to install a chemo port in our chest or arm.

After chemo, we lost the hair on our heads and all over our bodies. I felt like a hairless child, not a sexy woman. If we had nausea, mouth sores, or dry mouth, we had to forego kissing for a time. If we had neuropathy in our feet, we had to give up walking and exercising. We may have been swollen with edema. Many of us had gastrointestinal symptoms, always needing to be near a bathroom. If we had radiation, we needed to pull up our shirts and show our breasts, not only during treatment but regularly afterward to allow doctors or nurses to check the condition of our skin. The list of intrusions to privacy we suffered goes on and on.

I discovered the best way to get through it was to finally give in to the process, to relinquish control, and accept my situation. Yes, to surrender to it.

Learning to how to surrender, and being able to figure out just when to surrender, are valuable life skills. Accepting our loss of control and the inevitability of change can help us to cope with myriad other difficulties throughout our lives. We surrender when it's time to let our children grow up and leave us. We surrender when our parents and other loved ones die. We surrender when we look in the mirror and think, "Oh God, I've turned into my mother."

One of the most liberating realizations I can share with you is that I also learned to surrender my regrets. Last month I came across a letter that my mother wrote to me in 1990, two years after my father's death. As I read about the pleasure she took in fixing up a beautiful room for me when I was a little girl, I experienced a deep wave of regret. I regretted judging her for her drinking and her need to be the center of attention. Why had I focused so much on her limitations and not more on her genuine love for me? Why was I so unforgiving? What a terrible waste. She's been gone for fifteen years but I desperately wanted to ask her forgiveness. I wanted to tell her how much I loved her and to thank her for all she had done for me.

All I could do was talk to her in prayer and have faith that she heard me. I needed to surrender my regrets and be at peace with my own limitations, judgments, and imperfections. My mother would want this for me.

In my roles as a hospital chaplain and a hospice volunteer, I have stood by and comforted at least 200 people at their hour of death. Though each situation was different, I could not help but observe how many people died with a look of deep peace on their faces. These are people who have been able to surrender, find peace, and let go. As a friend half-jokingly said to me, "I can just let go when I die. I won't have to do my taxes, pay my bills, or deal with my ex." If our breast cancer can teach us the wondrous art of surrender, it will benefit us for the rest of our imperfect, unpredictable lives.

Questions for Reflection and Discussion

1. Are you a person who feels calmer when you have control?
2. If so, how did you react to turning over control to your medical team?
3. Can you see the benefits of sometimes surrendering in your own life? In what areas is this important for you now?
4. How do you think learning to surrender might help you and bring you peace?
5. What are you now trying to surrender?
6. What have you not yet tried to surrender, but need to?

Gift Five

SISTERHOOD

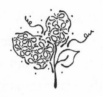

My sisters, recently I read a *New York Times* article entitled "What Women Find in Friends That They May Not Get From Love." The headline grabbed my attention because I could so easily relate. The support of other women was a lifesaver in my year of cancer. It has surprised and delighted me to see the beautiful outreach of not only my friends, but also relative strangers who heard of my illness. The positive energy from these women, the warm embrace of their care and concern for me, has helped me endure much anxiety and even to overcome outright fear.

Did you have a similar experience with the wonderful kindness of women in your life? Were they there for you during your time with breast cancer? Are they still?

I was not brought up to appreciate such kindness. We were a largely male clan. I had two brothers, but no sisters or female cousins. I grew up with neither grandmothers nor aunts in my life. The only significant female presence in my life was my mother, a woman who clearly preferred not to suffer the company of other women. She skipped out of women's groups in the church and the community. She never once in my memory invited ladies over for coffee and a chat. My mom was beautiful and flirtatious and had no problem indulging the attention of men, but she judged women to be competitive and untrustworthy.

In spite of this bias, she sent me to an all-girls Catholic high school that gave me at last, in addition to a fine education, exposure to the positive influence of many girls. It was in high school that I first realized that I needed girl-friends in my life. I remember going to Carol's house after school to drink Coke and watch *American Bandstand*. We danced and laughed and fantasized about the boys on the show and the romance between Justine and Bob. Carol took me in and treated me like a sister. She is still among my closest friends, although we live a thousand miles apart.

At my lowest point during chemo, two

other friends, Sue and Joyce, showed up at my house with armfuls of beautiful purple lilacs. Sue had prevailed through her own brief brush with breast cancer and had also undergone surgery for heart disease. Joyce lost her beloved husband, John, to liver cancer. These were friends who had walked through fire.

These women know the territory and know how to be truly present with someone who is struggling. "We thought you might need some hugs and sistering," Sue told me one day.

Did I ever! I was bald, sick, and scared. We sat in the family room where I had been sacked out under an afghan and I sobbed while they each held me. I told them that I was scared. I told them I doubted I could survive the treatment. My cardiac arrhythmia left me completely disabled at that time, unable to walk more than a few steps, and struggling for every breath.

Sue and Joyce were like mothers to me: listening, holding, understanding, and caring. I had similar experiences with so many other women. Some had been through the same ordeal or had suffered other health crises. Women rallied around in all the ways that mattered: bringing

food, sending flowers, writing cards both funny and sweet, dropping off uplifting novels, and
leaving supportive voice mails that I wasn't expected to return. The depth of their love was
amazing to me. I felt embarrassed, undeserving,
and humbled. I felt a bond with these women
that I knew would endure beyond my illness. I
discovered I had sisters after all.

What is it exactly that we receive from the
friendship of women? Why do we find it so sus-
taining? In my case, I felt from women the mir-
roring of my own complicated emotions, a sense
that they just "got it." I felt true empathy while
crying with my friends. I didn't need to explain to
them what I was going through—they just knew.

We are all in this beautiful, complicated life
together. None of us is so special that our life is
perfect. We can laugh at what a mess we are, or
how old we look, or how we screwed up again
with our kids. In my female friendships, I find
soothing acceptance, especially in times of crisis.

Of course, some women, like my mother,

aren't cut out to be that kind of friend. There are women who are competitive, and who prefer to maintain emotional distance. I have to admit that sometimes I feel jealous of younger or more attractive women, or feel sad that some women my age can still exercise in ways that my body can't manage anymore. But after experiencing such love and support from so many women, I decided I must in turn become this kind of friend for others.

Women have a knack for words. My female friends put words to feelings I wasn't truly conscious of and had never been able to voice. It was helpful beyond words to hear from one friend, "Wow, I'd be mad if that happened to me. Aren't you?"

With those words I felt at last the permission I so badly needed to fume about my breast cancer. To hear her speak aloud the words that I was silently muttering to myself helped immeasurably to dissipate any guilt I felt over being just plain mad.

I was especially blessed by the outreach of old friends. Were you too? An old, once very close, friend I hadn't seen in thirty years came for a visit. It felt so good to laugh with her again and remember the old boyfriends we each dated in grad school. It was such a relief to revel again in those happy times. Another friend sent me a beautiful hand-stitched quilt. Many friends put me on the prayer lists at their churches and regularly sent me encouraging—that is, giving courage—cards. One even enclosed a small red plastic heart to carry in my wallet to remind me of her prayers. Who but a woman would think of such a thing!

If I hadn't had breast cancer, I might have gone along in my life not fully realizing how much I was loved by my many "sisters." Such wonderful gifts we have to give one another, and how easily we find ways to give them. This new awareness of the power and importance of sisterhood has been a wonderful blessing in my life, and continues to motivate me to give back when the tables are turned. It is the singular force that motivated me to write this book.

Anaïs Nin said, "Each friend represents a world in us, a world not born until they arrive, and it is only by this meeting that a new world is born."

Questions for Reflection and Discussion

1. Who are your best friends? What do you love about them?
2. Do you now realize how much you mean to them?
3. Were women more precious to you during your breast cancer treatment than ever before? In what ways?
4. Are they still precious to you?
5. What exactly do you receive from your own "sisters"? Think about this in detail. Savor it.

Gift Six

NO LONGER NEEDING TO BE RIGHT

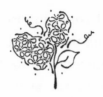

My sisters, picture this: I am five years old and a finalist in my kindergarten spelling bee. I know I can win; I'm a great speller. I'm given the word "bureau." I spell it "brereau," which is how I pronounce it. Just like that, I'm out. I'm mad, and convinced that the teacher is wrong. It's always been "brereau." It is so hard for me to accept that I am just plain wrong.

Recently I had a discussion with my son and daughter-in-law about whether my cardiac arrhythmia is inherited or not. I was convinced that it wasn't; they contended that it most likely was. At my next appointment, my cardiologist told me that it probably is inherited, so I went home, cut myself a big slice of humble pie and confessed my error. Admitting I was wrong was hard for me, but I came to realize that it actually served to strengthen my relationship with both my son and his wife.

As I age, I have begun to notice that I am wrong more often than I used to be. I find myself scribbling grocery and to-do lists now, and glancing surreptitiously at name tags at large social functions. Sometimes a word I've written just doesn't look right. Spellcheck is helpful, but I'd rather have the brain I had in my twenties.

Just recently, I said to my husband, "I'd like to drive west to see those presidents who are carved into that mountain. What's it called?"

It took me ten minutes to come up with Mt. Rushmore.

Watching helplessly while my father, and then my brother, developed dementia compounded my anxiety. The relentless progression of that disease was truly terrifying. The likelihood that I may have some "chemo brain" or "chemo fog," and not dementia, has helped to calm my jittery nerves. My oncologist assures me that the harmful effects of chemotherapy on cognition can last for years. She also graciously mentioned that although she is only fifty, she often forgets a word too.

Are such fears affecting you, despite the reassurance of your doctor? Do you find yourself in error more often than you'd like? Does it scare you as it scares me? Chemo brain is one of the more difficult side effects of our cancer treatment.

Just as the toxic drugs circulating in our bodies kill the cancer cells, they kill healthy cells everywhere. That's why we develop side effects that are so often highly visible: hair loss, weight loss or weight gain, edema, rashes, just to name a few. The physical changes in our brains, while not visible, are just as real and even more troubling.

Dr. Carolyn Kaelin discusses brain changes related to cancer treatment in her book, *Living Through Breast Cancer*. Changes, she writes, may include:

- *Difficulty concentrating or paying attention, especially when multitasking*
- *Slowed ability to process information*
- *Trouble learning and remembering new information*
- *Trouble recalling words*
- *Losing one's train of thought midsentence*
- *Increased forgetfulness*

- *Difficulty remembering planned events*
- *Difficulty interpreting and recalling visual patterns*
- *Decreased mental flexibility so that small, unanticipated changes seem overwhelming*

Dr. Kaelin cautions that for some women these changes may be short-lived but for others they can last a decade. No one can tell us definitively whether these changes are caused exclusively by chemo or are a result of chemo in combination with other factors that may include aging, poor sleep, general fatigue, or other meds we may be taking. These mental changes affect nearly all cancer patients and for some reason are rarely talked about.

In my experience, a combination of patience and humor can make an enormous difference. I may not be able to hurry the recovery process, but I can laugh at my mistakes—at least on a good day. My husband and I have developed a betting system to lighten the situation. We call it our "You Owe Me a Quarter" solution. When a disagreement on a point of fact arises, whoever is proven wrong has to cough up a quarter.

So far, I'm only down fifty cents.

Suffering from an overabundance of pride in always being right is a tough way to go through life. Because I was successful as a student, I got into the habit of assuming that I knew better than everyone else. In a funny way, it feels like a relief to give that up. Being wrong no longer shatters my self-esteem. I just hand over the quarter.

In Lisa Genova's bestselling novel *Still Alice*, the main character, who suffers from dementia, remains her lovable self despite her mental decline. Although she can no longer express herself the way she used to, she still feels all the feelings, and lives the full life, of a loving and empathetic mother.

Those of us struggling with cognitive issues related to chemo need to remember that, even if a word escapes us, it doesn't mean we are suffering from dementia. It isn't permanent. And it doesn't make us any less valuable, less loving, or less lovable.

My family history of cognitive decline due to neurodegenerative illness has made my own mental slips very scary. Maybe you also have had these concerns. For me, humor and self-compassion have been fabulous antidotes to anxiety. I remain at heart undiminished by these little slips. I am no less myself because of them. I am still Kay.

And I am learning, despite my ingrained inclination to the contrary, that not having to be right all the time is a blessing. Letting go of that need can significantly reduce the fear of cognitive decline as we age. Whatever the past has brought us and whatever the future holds, cancer treatment has given us coping tools. I hope that you, my sisters, will also see the blessing in not having to be right.

Just be sure to have some quarters handy.

Questions for Reflection and Discussion

1. Have you had more difficulty remembering things since your treatment? Talk about that.
2. Has it been frustrating? Even scary? What do you fear?
3. Have you had the experience of caring for or helping someone who has experienced cognitive loss? How did you manage that? How does that help you with your own mental slips.
4. Do you find that you can sometimes laugh at your mistakes? Can you give an example?
5. Or do you fear that your brain will never return to the way it was?
6. What can you do to relieve yourself of this anxiety?

Gift Seven

SAVORING EACH DAY

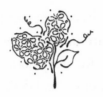

My sisters, the first spring after completing my cancer treatment was the most beautiful spring that I can remember. Just outside my window, the lilacs exploded into bloom. Have they always, I wonder, exuded such a glorious fragrance? I noticed the splash of rain on the sidewalk. Has it always sounded so musical? Why then, did I not have the ears to hear it? I was happy to be alive.

Did you also experience a swell of relief and pleasure upon ending your treatment? Did you feel you had turned a page in your life, as I did? Cancer is a watershed event in our lives; there is the "before," and there is the "since," and they are two very different worlds.

Serious illness can teach us, if we only will listen, to appreciate every day we have. We may grieve and fear recurrence, but there is also deep joy in being alive—right here, right now. I feel a special pleasure this moment in the hot mug of coffee that I always keep at hand when I am writing. I feel pleasure in seeing the little kids arriving at the library for story hour, their faces glowing with excitement. I feel delight in taking long walks and noticing the subtle daily changes in my neighborhood. I've been watching a house being built, measuring the daily progress and marveling at the miracle of craftsmen and craftswomen building someone not just a new house but a new home. If you look closely, there are changes every day in everything around us. As Heraclitus told us twenty-five centuries ago: "No man ever steps in the same river twice, for it's not the same river and he's not the same man." How true I find that to be. How much I have changed. I now feel more present than I ever have been in my daily life. I am following the advice of the poet Mary Oliver, who urges us to value this one "wild and precious" life. The Persian poet and mystic Rumi beautifully reminds us that "when you do things from your soul, you feel a river moving in you, a joy."

Nature beckons and calls us to attention. Is that an indigo bunting perched on that tree? Is that maple dancing, shimmering in the breath of a light summer breeze?

I was driving down a highway with a friend, a talented graphic designer, one gloomy day late in autumn, when she remarked, to my surprise, "What beautiful colors." I opened my eyes then, to what was right in front of me, and saw not just a tired display of grays and tans, but a wide palette of ochers and umbers and raspberry hues everywhere along the roadside. I have been able to see them ever since. I also see decaying trees and wilting flowers now and realize that life is an ongoing process of growth and decline, life and death. I have come to appreciate that this cycle unavoidably includes me. My own mortality finally registers amid my frantic attempts to make myself look younger and the wacky fallacy that I have all the time in the world. The shock of cancer has taught me that I truly have only today.

The sense that we are all in this together is a great consolation and increases my empathy for everyone I meet. Everyone is my sister or brother and all of us must suffer, if not now then later. We are simultaneously fragile and strong. The lives we live are over-brimming with incredible beauty if only we can find the eyes to behold it.

The human family in all its diversity charms me now in a way it never did before my illness. I feel connected with everyone I see. I am at our local library and this is what I see: a three-year-old with sparkling shoes dancing by with her pony-tailed mother; a bent, gray-haired man outside checking under the hood of his Camry, tinkering patiently; a care-free back-packed student sauntering by, hands in his jeans pockets, singing a quiet song to himself; a dad with three books ambling by while his much taller son stares at his smart phone. The human family is so beautiful in its diversity, and I now bear full witness to that beauty.

For some time after my mother's death, it felt like my brain just stopped working. I couldn't remember my own phone number for a week or two and the names of people I knew perfectly well eluded me. My grief expressed itself cognitively as well as emotionally. At the same time, I was startled to hear birdsongs that I had never heard before. My hearing was amplified and sharpened. I became acutely aware of the inevitable fact that I too will die someday. The shock of her sudden death gave me pause to consider the certainty of my own inevitable mortality.

Cancer has affected me in the same way. Maybe it has been this way for you, too. We may feel freer to live the life we want and to stop judging ourselves for our mistakes. I notice that I spend money a little more freely; I eat more slowly, savoring each bite, instead of rushing through the paper while I breakfast. I listen to my body saying, "Just go outside and enjoy a good walk, and skip the rigors of the health club for today." Although I weigh myself every day, I can more easily forgive a couple of pounds resulting from that pizza with everything or that lavish dinner out. I just shrug my shoulders now, and plan a salad for my next meal.

Recently, I bought an outrageously over-priced lipstick I'd been eager to try. Was it worth it? The old me would have said, "No way." But it is creamy and lovely and I feel like a queen wearing it. So yes, it's worth it. What or who am I saving my money for? Like the old song says, my children, God bless them, have got their own. While most of my wardrobe remains budget friendly (who doesn't love Kohl's cash!), I might now splurge on an occasional trip to Nordstrom.

I donate more money to charities, too, and enjoy doing it, choosing carefully those that matter the most to me.

Surviving chemo has even enhanced my already healthy and life-long love of good books. During treatment, I felt almost addicted to reading. It was a wonderful distraction from my heart problems, my fatigue, the taste of metal in my mouth, and my worry. I continue to enjoy books now more than ever. I also enjoy writing, putting my deepest thoughts out there with the fervent hope that they will resonate with someone, and that they will help make someone's life better in some way.

Your experience may not resemble mine, but I trust that some part of this book will help you—as this whole experience has helped me— to live life more fully. Connecting with you, my sisters, is another way I'm savoring every day.

Questions for Reflection and Discussion

1. Are you able to enjoy one day at a time more than you used to?

2. What small pleasures do you savor? What gives you joy? Explain.

3. Do you now have greater awareness of your mortality?

4. If so, has that depressed you? Frightened you? Talk about that.

5. Or has coming to terms with death made each day more precious? In what ways?

Gift Eight

DISCOVERING YOUR OWN STRENGTH AND BEAUTY

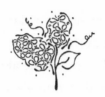

My sisters, it is a golden September day in 1950. I'm a little girl in a blue dress, long blonde hair, slightly chubby, and I've just started first grade. I struggle on my trip home to walk up Governor Long Road, which is no more than a hill, really, but today looms like a mountain before me.

As I collapse into an easy chair at home I gasp, "I can't breathe, Mommy."

Pulling air in, pushing it out, over and over. My heart pounds. I'm scared and gasping for breath.

My mom leans over me, frowning with concern and bewilderment. "What's wrong, honey? What's wrong?"

Later, she tells my dad, "Kay couldn't get up the hill without gasping for breath. I think she needs to see the doctor."

I am diagnosed with asthma and begin a six-month regimen of allergy shots. Once a week at seven in the evening my dad drives me to the doctor. I remember to this day how much I enjoyed our brief but rare time alone together.

I was disturbed one evening to overhear the doctor tell my father, in a hushed tone, "She may never be able to run. A condition like hers doesn't just go away."

This is the first time I discovered that my body had limitations, that I couldn't always rely on it to do what I wanted it to do. If I had been diagnosed today, my asthma would have been better managed. But treatment was limited at that time. The condition was poorly understood, and sometimes treated as if it were nothing more than a cry for attention. As a child, I felt confused and ashamed of my limitations. Because kids assumed I couldn't run, I was usually picked near last for gym teams. I remember so well the feeling of humiliation standing against the wall as the line of girls dwindled. I remained chubby until puberty, when I grew tall and finally lost the baby fat.

I share this story now to show how much of a struggle I have had coming to appreciate my lovely, healthy body. I have been fortunate to have lived free of illness until these past few years, though my asthma does still prevent me from engaging in strenuous exercise. I sometimes drop out in the middle of the seniors' exercise class because I have trouble breathing. It makes me feel like I'm six years old again, ashamed, and sad.

Paradoxically, the diagnosis of breast cancer has helped me learn to accept my physical limitations. I am thankful for the good health I do have. Just as nobody is perfect, few are in perfect health. What I am is good enough.

This same spirit of acceptance can also apply to sex. It doesn't have to be fabulous to be good. Caressing can feel more loving than orgasm. Struggling with illness and a changed body as a result of that illness can make us feel less desirable. This is bound to complicate our sexual relations. When orgasm is frustratingly elusive, I often think of the comedian Wanda Sykes' hilarious line, "Hey, this time the train ain't leavin' the station."

Letting go of the pressure for perfection can make sex much more pleasurable. Good enough is okay for now.

Illness can mature us. Do you sense that too? Now that we are scarred by breast cancer and our bodies no longer look the way they once did, we can either endlessly grieve over our lost past self or grow to accept being the person we are today. Our lives are always in transition; we get older and change every day.

My vibrantly alive eighty-year-old friend Helen expressed it this way: "Every day when I wake up I ask myself, 'Okay what hurts today?' And I laugh or I groan. What can you do? It's life, dang it!"

You may have guessed it: Helen is also a breast cancer survivor.

Our souls are forged by the refining fire of illness. It is just another respect in which cancer gives us a gift. Perfectionism is out, contentment is in. It is a gift to be resilient in the face of grief and loss and to rejoice just in being alive.

Questions for Reflection and Discussion

1. How has breast cancer changed your view of yourself?
2. Do you feel less desirable now?
3. Are romantic relationships more challenging? Talk about that.
4. Are you able to love your body just as it is right now?
5. What would help you accept the changes you see?
6. If you've lost a breast or two breasts, how have you dealt with that loss?
7. Do you believe that cancer has matured you? In what ways?
8. Do you feel more resilient than you were?

Gift Nine

DEEPER SPIRITUALITY

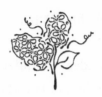

My sisters, our lives are made up of equal parts sorrow and joy and we are well designed to withstand both. Cancer awakens us—there is nothing like a brush with death to startle the spirit into seeing the gorgeousness of life. Cancer awakened in me an infinitely more spiritual nature.

Spirituality is a deep awareness of the divinity infusing all things: in the man and woman in the Honda at the stoplight, in grass and weeds, in stars and planets, even in our beloved pets. All things that breathe: hollyhocks, lilacs, daisies, exotic indigo buntings, ordinary red-breasted robins, a mangy hyena, a magnificent panther—all are filled with breath and therefore spirit.

Spirituality is also the realization that our lives have a deeper meaning than what is on the surface. Spirituality makes us ask ourselves serious questions about our lives. Why am I here? What is my life about? What am I supposed to be doing with my life? What can I leave behind when I die?

It's a good idea to differentiate between spirituality and religion. For many, conventional religiosity supports their spirituality very well. Others feel that even though they may think of themselves as deeply spiritual they are not expressly religious. This attitude can be the result of a negative experience with organized religion, or a just a wish to be free from creeds and clerics. Religious doctrines of all sorts muddy the waters when they insist we follow their one, approved way to achieve spiritual depth.

For me, religious faith has greatly enhanced my spirituality by encouraging me to look ever more deeply into the meaning of my life, by giving me stories and examples to reflect about, by raising questions that I feel free to ponder. Cancer reminded me of the preciousness of life. To remain mindful of that preciousness is a beautiful gift. After the grief and fear, the pain and loss, there is beauty in just being alive, in having survived.

It is a lovely warm October evening in 1978. My husband Phil and I have just left the house for a much-needed weekend away in Wisconsin. Our eight-year-old son and six-year-old daughter are with a friend. I am three months pregnant and thrilled about it. As we drive, I feel the need to use a restroom, so we stop at a gas station and I notice a spot of blood. Back in the car I mention this but remain relaxed and happy to be getting away.

After checking into Lake Lawn Lodge, we go out to dinner and I order a steak, which I eat with gusto. After dinner, I stop to use the ladies' room and suddenly blood pours out of me in a frightening rush. I manage to clean up and somehow walk back to the table, sit down and pass out. My husband calls our waitress who brings me a wheelchair and calls 911. I am hardly aware of where I am.

At the hospital, I'm told that I have had a miscarriage and that I'll need a D&C. As I am wheeled into surgery, an amazingly tender anesthesiologist calms me with his presence, smile, and gentle words. Because of him, I have a deep sense that I am in God's hands.

◇ ◇ ◇ ◇ ◇

In the following weeks, I found myself walking through a gray fog. I felt the loss of the child acutely. I remember mundane moments, such as putting gas in my car, thinking that I'd never been so sad. I'd wanted that baby so much.

I believe that many spiritual experiences happen principally through the goodness of other people, especially during painful times. A higher power exists in the beauty of another's care and concern for us. When we most need them, others help us find our way. Albert Schweitzer, theologian and philosopher, said, "At times our own light goes out and is rekindled by a spark from another person."

Spirituality can also help to make sense of our feelings: frustrated longings, deep grief, sudden sorrow, regret, guilt, or anger. Spirituality can help us see how even painful experiences dovetail with the rest of our lives.

Spiritual reading and reflection can also help, especially when we are feeling lost and alone. Some passages that helped me find myself again when I felt lost:

Reinhold Niebuhr's Serenity Prayer: *God, grant me the serenity to accept the things I cannot change; courage to change the things I can, and wisdom to know the difference. Living one day at a time, Enjoying one moment at a time, Accepting hardship as a pathway to peace....*

Psalm 23:4: *Even though I walk through the valley of the shadow of death, I will fear no evil, for you are with me; your rod and your staff comfort me.*

Psalm 91:3: *He will rescue you from the fowler's snare, from the destroying plague....*

Psalm 138:7: *Though I walk in the midst of dangers, you guard my life when my enemies rage. You stretch out your hand; your right hand saves me.*

And the wonderful Gospel of John 14:1, 27: *Do not let your hearts be troubled.... Peace I leave with you; my peace I give to you.*

Questions for Reflection and Discussion

1. Do you sometimes wonder why you are here?
2. Who or what has helped you with this? Describe this person or experience.
3. Do you need someone to talk to about this aspect of your life?
4. Has religion been a help or a hindrance to you in sorting this out? Explain.
5. Do you have a fundamental belief in the value and meaning of your life? Elaborate please.

OPENING THE NINE GIFTS

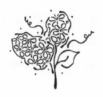

My sisters, we have come a long way. Our hearts, minds, and spirits are in a different place because of our walk with breast cancer. We are wiser now. We know that we can't control everything. We know that life is unpredictable. How do we make the most of our new wisdom and awareness? How do we best unwrap the gifts we have been given? Some of these discoveries, like my new awareness, and acceptance, of interdependence, are complicated by many years of habit and attitude. Even the new me must admit that trying to laugh when I am wrong still causes me anxiety and embarrassment.

After fighting cancer, all of us need a large dose of self-compassion. Self-compassion lies at the foundation of our healing. Without it, we will struggle to "get over" what has happened to us. It's tempting to go back to our old habits, pushing cancer out of our minds as though it's all behind us. But we need to recognize that we are fundamentally changed. Our attitudes need adjustment as well. Ask yourself:

- Have I learned to focus more on the things that I enjoy?
- Am I paying greater attention to how I am feeling and what I need for the day? Not necessarily what I need *to do*, but what do my body, heart, and mind need to flourish today?
- Do I remember now to treat myself as I would treat someone I dearly love?

When I retired from my psychology practice, I knew I wanted to write. I had already made a habit of writing regularly, but that effort was limited to daily journal entries. Cancer encouraged me to reach beyond the "Dear Diary" construct. Although it's scary somedays to face the blank page or screen, it is also fun to see the words that spill out. I struggle with doubt, questioning whether it's all been said before by someone far more articulate than I am. But I trust in my heart that *we each have a story to tell* and that there is great value in sharing them. I love to read other people's stories. I learn from them and enjoy being let into their lives.

Living through cancer can stimulate our creativity by giving us permission to do more of what we want. I recently gave a friend a mug that says, "Do more of what makes you happy." I am determined now to take those words to heart myself.

One thing that I have learned through my whole ordeal is that I need a place of refuge, a place where I can be completely alone and at peace. My refuge is usually a corner of the sofa in our family room. In the quiet hours of early morning, I sit there with my mug of coffee and my journal. In the afternoon, I like to read there. I also go there to pray every day.

Where is your place of refuge, the spot you have carved out for yourself? It may be a physical place or even just an internal space that you retreat to in your mind. For others, it's a favorite vacation spot. Many of us crave being outdoors, finding that nature has healing power. It doesn't matter where our refuge is, only that we allow ourselves to be there and enjoy it, that we remain mindful of it, and take ourselves there with regularity. Feeling peace and joy is essential for our healing.

Our eating, exercise patterns, and even breathing may also change after our experience with cancer. Relaxation is crucial to recovery. Because of my asthma history, I have worked hard on breathing more deeply. Mindful breathing and meditation calm both my mind and my body. It's the best medicine there is for me.

What is the best medicine for you? Maybe it's laughter, dancing, swimming, or singing. Whatever it is, give yourself permission to do more of it. Open the gift of your personal joy— and do it every day.

Another way to appreciate the gifts that cancer can bring is by being an active part of a community that increases your happiness. Feeling free to say, "No, that won't work for me" frees us to say, "Yes, sign me up" to something you really want to do.

For the past four years, I have co-led a book discussion group. About twenty of us meet every Thursday morning to discuss a book and share whatever thoughts and feelings the book has stimulated in us. We started with Joan Chittister's *The Gift of Years*, which was very meaningful to all of us, and we have gone on to many other books. But since my experience with cancer, I have noticed that my enthusiasm for leading the group has waned. I've decided to step down, something I never would have empowered myself to do before I had cancer. The group will most likely benefit from having a new leader, someone who brings *her* energy to something she is truly called to do.

This past holiday season, I got involved in a gift drive through my local church. A large group convened to load a semi with hundreds of items that had been collected for struggling families. It was freezing outside and snow was expected. Excited teenagers had gathered, blowing on their hands to keep warm. The pastor opened with a prayer, someone turned on Brenda Lee's swinging rendition of "Rockin' Around the Christmas Tree" and the work began. We formed a long line made up of little kids, seniors, teens, married couples, singles, widows, and widowers.

Our leader shouted directions, "No kid should pick up a box larger than this one! Don't hurt your back—ask for help with heavy boxes! Stay in line, we can do this!"

I was thrilled, smiling, dancing to the music, and loving this sense of shared purpose. Tears came to my eyes seeing the excitement in the little kids as they wheeled bikes for less fortunate children into the trailer. The teens, too, loved being useful; they poured out their abundant energy. The bigger men stood at the back of the truck and passed everything up. After the truck was fully loaded, we collectively exhaled with pleasure. It was a job well done, and we had done it together. This simple event embodied the meaning of Christmas for me. Together we had achieved something larger than ourselves.

Being part of a community and making a contribution to society is energizing. We all have unique gifts to share and a role to play here on earth. The new awareness we have about the vulnerability of our lives gives us a fresh perspective—one that we ought to share with others. We don't rush through life so hurriedly. We notice the world unfurling around us more. We want to do whatever good is ours to do today. We now know that we don't have forever; we only have now. Whether it's a smile I give to the checkout girl or the compliment I share with a stranger, small gestures make the world a friendlier place.

You may wonder how to do this if you are still struggling with sadness, fear, or anger. Fear of recurrence threatens to flatten us with every mammogram or medical test. Those are the moments when self-compassion can come to our rescue. We need to stop for just a moment, and remember to be kind to ourselves. As a cancer survivor, whether you are still in treatment or in remission, you are a shining light of wisdom in a death-denying culture. Live fully each moment, knowing it's all we really have. What a gift you are! Enjoy the beautiful new you. You, my sisters, are a blessing to this world.

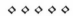

Questions for Reflection and Discussion

1. Are you kinder to yourself than you used to be? In what ways?
2. Do you see the value in self-compassion? Elaborate on this.
3. What gives you joy? Describe it.
4. Do you realize how precious you are?

ACKNOWLEDGMENTS

Bringing a book to life is a process requiring deep faith that the work is valuable and many helpers to attend the birth. I am very grateful to have had wonderful editing by Michael Coyne at In Extenso Press, and the beautiful creative work by designer Patricia Lynch. I am also grateful to Greg Pierce of ACTA Publications who referred me to Mike as the best person to edit this particular manuscript.

Bill O'Hanlon's on-line writing course gave me the initial inspiration to write my story and Nora Walsh Kerr's suggestions on the text were crucial in getting me going. My women's groups, which contain many breast cancer survivors, spurred me on.

I want to thank the medical teams at North Shore University Health Systems for getting me through four surgeries, chemo, and radiation and supporting me emotionally all the way.

And my wonderful internist, Dr. Janet Barczyk, whom I have leaned on for thirty years, was my rock, reminding me not to get ahead of myself when I was scared.

My family also played a big part: my son Phil, a much-published writer himself, cheered me on. My daughter Katherine gave me valuable help with complementary medicine. And my son David, knowing that nothing delights me like the grandchildren, regularly sent me texted photos of his two-year-old twins. Made me grin every time!

And the unfailing support and love of my husband Phil—well, there are just no words.

SUGGESTED RESOURCES
FOR FURTHER READING

Alschuler, Lisa. *The Definitive Guide to Thriving After Cancer.* NY: Ten Speed Press, 2013.

Andrew, Elizabeth. *Writing the Sacred Journey: The Art and Practice of Spiritual Memoir.* Boston: Skinner House Books, 2005.

Armstrong, Karen. *Twelve Steps to a Compassionate Life.* NY: Alfred Knopf, 2010.

Barks, Coleman with Moyne, John, translations. *The Essential Rumi.* San Francisco: Harper Collins, 1996.

Breathnach, Sarah Ben. *Simple Abundance: A Daybook of Comfort and Joy.* NY: Warner Books, 1995.

Cain, Susan. *Quiet: The Power of Introverts in a World that Can't Stop Talking.* NY: Crown, 2012

Carr, Kris. *Crazy Sexy Cancer Tips.* Guilford, CT: Morris Publishing, 2007.

Chittister, Joan. *The Sacred In-Between: Spiritual Wisdom for Life's Every Moment.* New London, CT: Twenty-Third Publications, 2013.

Dreamer, Oriah Mountain. *The Dance: Moving to the Rhythms of Your True Self.* NY: Harper Collins, 2001.

Hoffman, Alice. *Survival Lessons.* Chapel Hill, NC: Algonquin Books. 2013.

Kaelin, Carolyn. *Living Through Breast Cancer.* Cambridge, MA: McGraw Hill, 2005.

Kurtz, Ernest and Ketcham, Katherine. *The Spirituality of Imperfection: Story Telling and the Search for Meaning.* US: Bantam, 1992

Mendes, Dena. *A Survivor's Guide to Kicking Cancer's Ass.* US: Hay House, 2011.

Merrill, Nan. *Psalms for Praying: An Invitation to Wholeness.* NY: Continuum International Publishing Group: 1996.

Northrup, Christine. *Women's Bodies, Women's Wisdom,* Revised. NY: Bantam, 2010.

Novy-Bennewitz, Cara. *Diagnosis: Breast Cancer: The Best Action Plan for Navigating Your Journey.* Rolling Meadows, IL: Windy City Publications, 2012.

O'Regan, Ruth, et al. *Breast Cancer Journey: The Essential Guide to Treatment and Recovery.* Third Edition. Atlanta, GA: American Cancer Society, 2013.

Sheehy, Sandy. *Connecting: The Enduring Power of Female Friendship.* NY: Harper Collins, 2000.

Silver, Julie. *Chicken Soup for the Soul: Hope and Healing for Your Breast Cancer Journey.* Cos Cob, CT: Simon and Schuster, 2012.

Simmons, Philip. *Learning to Fall: The Blessings of an Imperfect Life*. NY: Bantam, 2000.

Silverman, Dan and Davidson, Idelle. *Your Brain After Chemo: A Practical Guide to Lifting the Fog and Getting Back Your Focus*. Cambridge, MA: Da Capo Press. 2009.

Taylor, Barbara Brown. *Learning to Walk in the Dark*. NY: Harper Collins, 2016.

Traister, Rebecca. "What Women Find in Friends That They May Not Get From Love," *New York Times*, Op-Ed, Sunday Review, Feb. 28, 2016.

Wicks, Robert J. *Spiritual Resilience: Thirty Days to Refresh Your Soul*. Cincinnati, OH: Franciscan Media, 2015.

Wiederkehr, Macrina. *Seasons of Your Heart*. NJ: Silver Burdette, 1979.

Other Books from In Extenso Press

ALL THINGS TO ALL PEOPLE: A Catholic Church for the Twenty-First Century, by Louis DeThomasis, FSC, 118 pages, paperback

CATHOLIC BOY BLUES: A Poet's Journey of Healing,
by Norbert Krapf, 224 pages, paperback

CATHOLIC WATERSHED: The Chicago Ordination Class of 1969 and How They Helped Change the Church,
by Michael P. Cahill, 394 pages, paperback

CHRISTIAN CONTEMPLATIVE LIVING:
Six Connecting Points, by Thomas M. Santa, CSSR, 126 pages, paperback

GREAT MEN OF THE BIBLE: A Guide for Guys,
by Martin Pable, OFM Cap, 216 pages, paperback

THE GROUND OF LOVE AND TRUTH: Reflections on Thomas Merton's Relationship with the Woman Known as "M,"
by Suzanne Zuercher, OSB, 120 pages, paperback

HOPE: One Man's Journey of Discovery from Tormented Child to Social Worker to Spiritual Director, by Marshall Jung, 172 pages, paperback

MASTER OF CEREMONIES: A Novel,
by Donald Cozzens, 288 pages, paperback and hardcover

NAVIGATING ALZHEIMER'S: 12 Truths about Caring for Your Loved One,
by Mary K. Doyle, 112 pages, paperback

PISTACO: A Tale of Love in the Andes,
by Lynn F. Monahan, 298 pages, paperback and hardcover-

SHRINKING THE MONSTER: Healing the Wounds of Our Abuse,
by Norbert Krapf, 234 pages, paperback

THE SILENT SCHISM: Healing the Serious Split in the Catholic Church,
by Louis DeThomasis, FSC, and Cynthia A. Nienhaus, CSA, 128 pages, paperback

THE UNPUBLISHED POET: On Not Giving Up on Your Dream,
by Marjorie L. Skelly, 160 pages, paperback

WAYWARD TRACKS: Revelations about fatherhood, faith, fighting with your spouse, surviving Girl Scout camp…, by Mark Collins, 104 pages, paperback

WE THE (LITTLE) PEOPLE, artwork by ISz, 50 plates, paperback

YOUR SECOND TO LAST CHAPTER: Creating a Meaningful Life on Your Own Terms, by Paul Wilkes, 120 pages, paperback and hardcover

BAPTIZED FOR THIS MOMENT: Rediscovering Grace All Around Us,
by Stephen Paul Bouman, 168 pages, paperback

AVAILABLE FROM BOOKSELLERS
OR FROM 800-397-2282 • INEXTENSOPRESS.COM
DISTRIBUTED EXCLUSIVELY BY ACTA PUBLICATIONS

Advance Praise for *After the Fear*

As a cancer survivor, I found myself responding "yes" over and over again to Kay's reflections on her own journey with this life-changing disease. How I wish I would have had the benefit of her wisdom as an anchor and a guide when I was in the midst of the storm.

— Chaplain Bob Backis, BCC

Kay's journey eloquently summarizes what so many of my patients with serious illness struggle with. After reading *After the Fear Come the Gifts*, I have a better understanding of what my patients are going through. This has helped me approach patients differently. I have been able to focus more on their emotional and psychological needs, which often times get buried in the management of pressing medical needs.

— Dr. Janet Barczyk, MD